A is for Autism

by

Jennifer Bloink

© 2005 Jennifer Bloink. All Rights Reserved.

No part of this book may be reproduced, stored in a retrieval system, or transmitted by any means without the written permission of the author.

First published by AuthorHouse 04/08/05

ISBN: 1-4208-4463-6 (sc)

Printed in the United States of America
Bloomington, Indiana

This book is printed on acid-free paper.

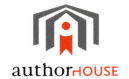

authorHOUSE

1663 LIBERTY DRIVE
BLOOMINGTON, INDIANA 47403
(800) 839-8640
www.authorhouse.com

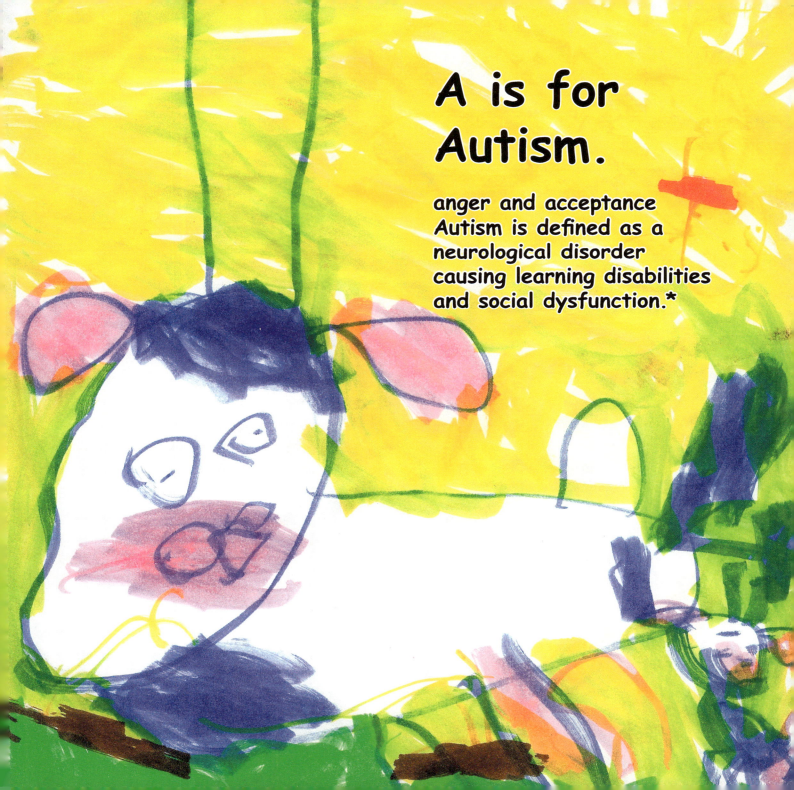

A is for Autism.

anger and acceptance
Autism is defined as a neurological disorder causing learning disabilities and social dysfunction.*

B is for Boy.

Occurence is twice as high in boys than in girls.*

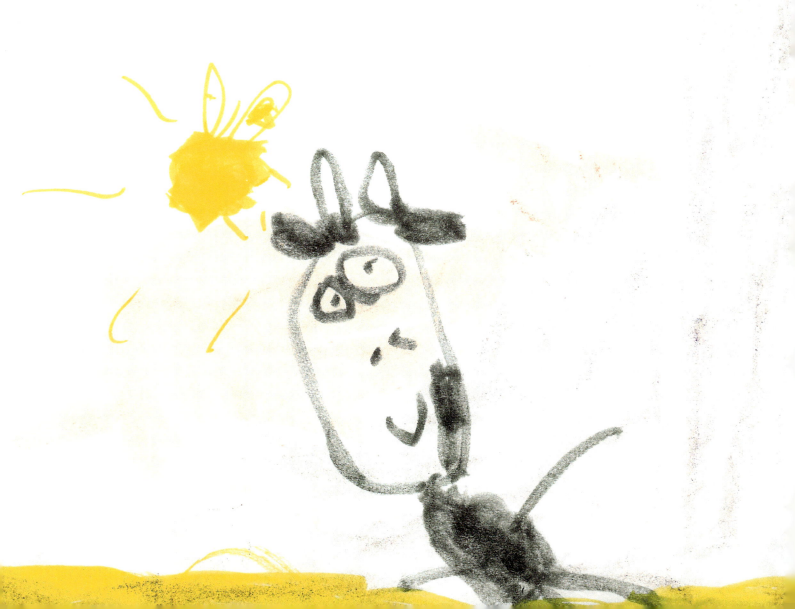

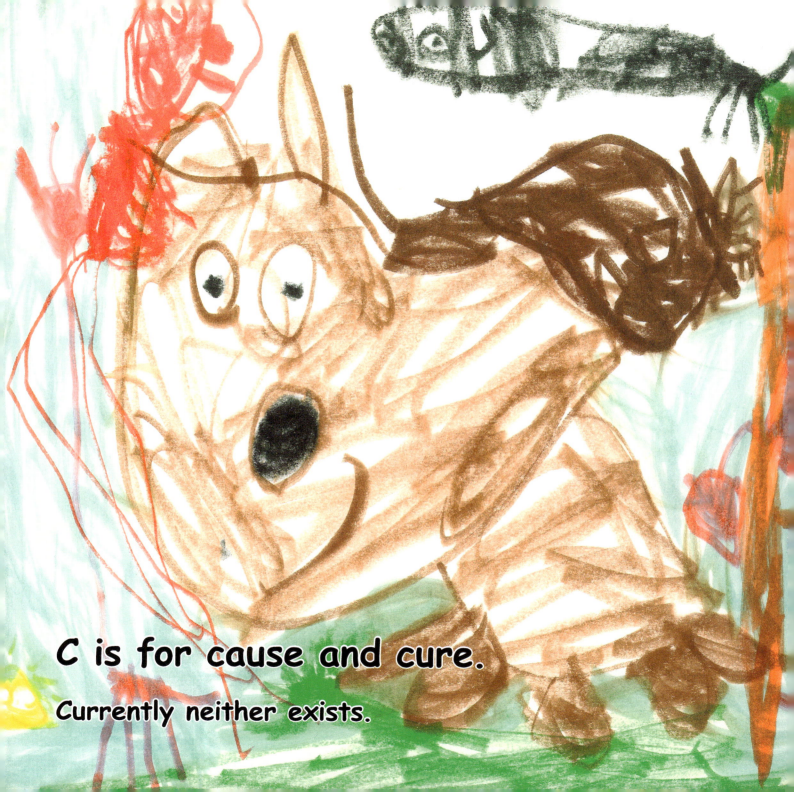

C is for cause and cure.

Currently neither exists.

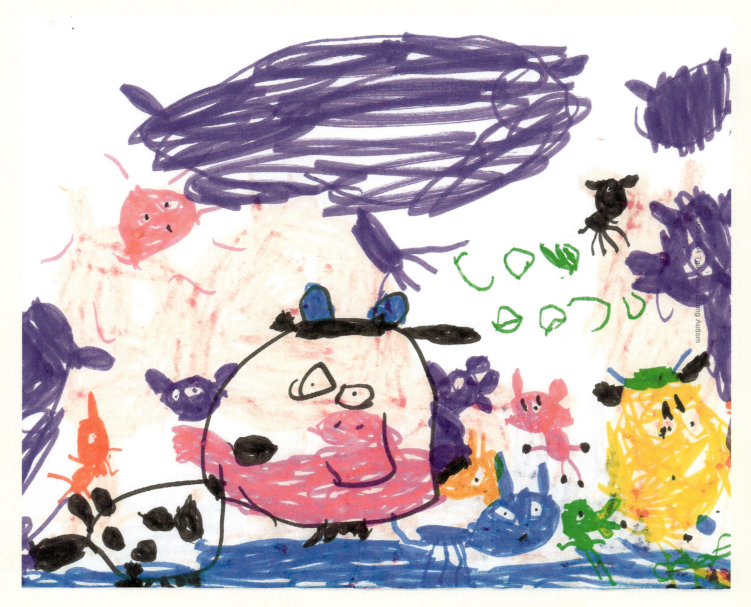

D is for Drugs and DON'T.

And discipline - autistic behavior is **not** a discipline problem.

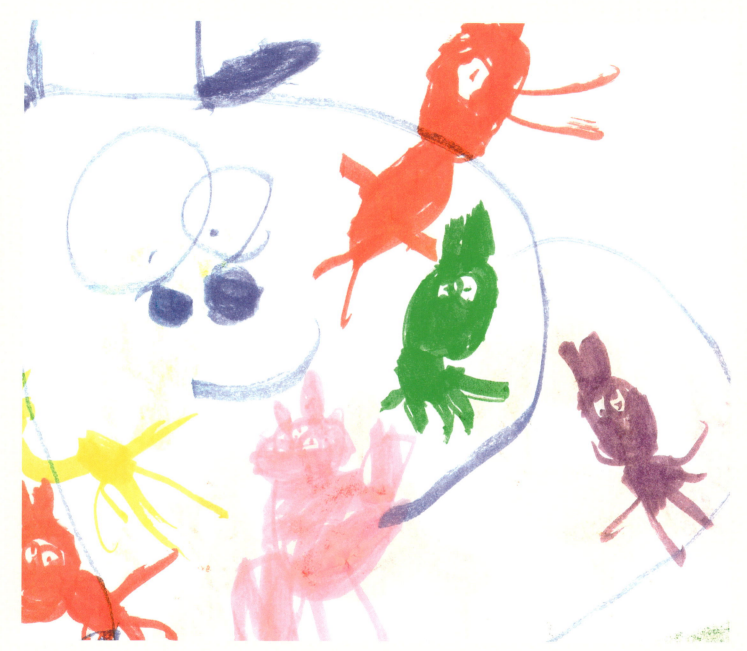

E is for education - for everyone.

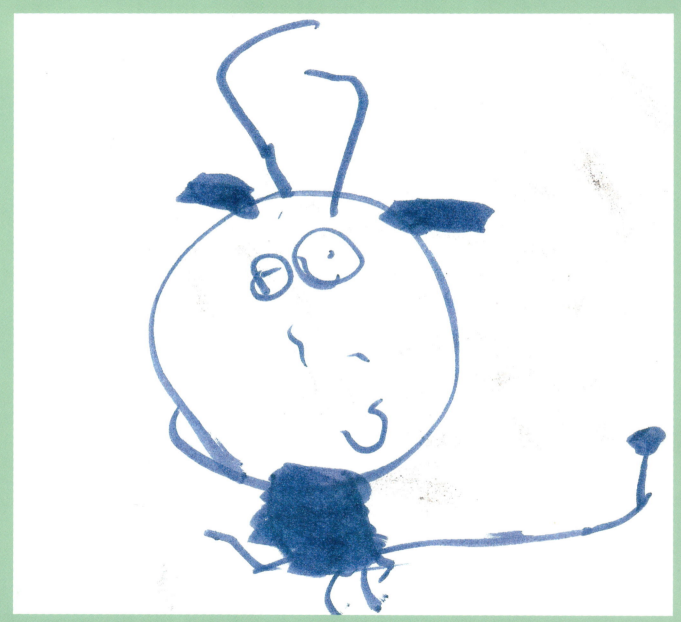

F is for future - also for everyone.

G is GFCF (gluten-free/casein-free).

Gluten is an enzyme in wheat; casein is an enzyme in dairy. The first step in the autism diet is to eliminate wheat and dairy. A complete allergy panel is advised.

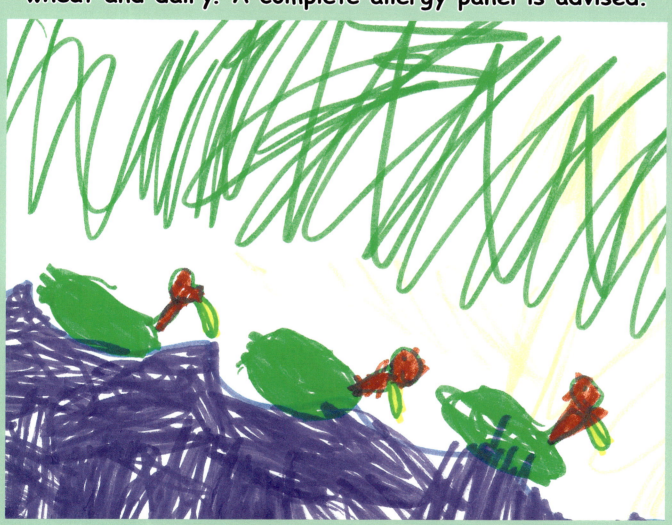

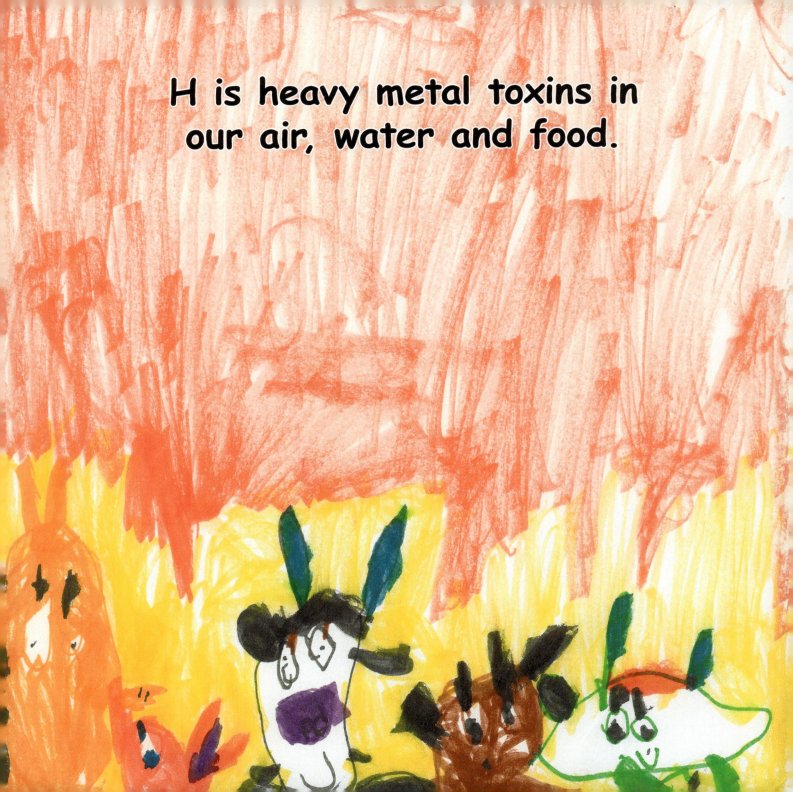
H is heavy metal toxins in our air, water and food.

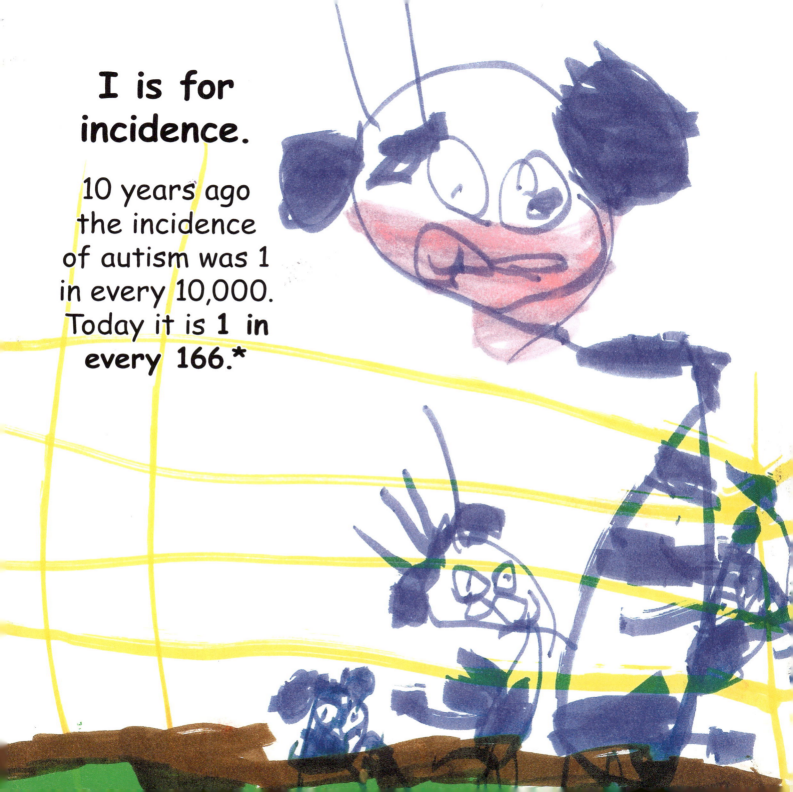

I is for incidence.

10 years ago the incidence of autism was 1 in every 10,000. Today it is **1 in every 166.***

J is for justice.

Keep voting for special education and children's rights.

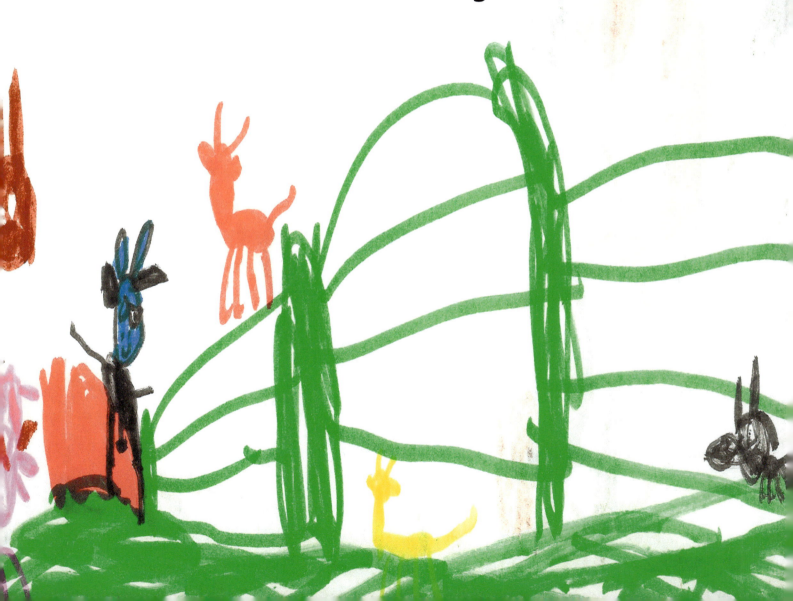

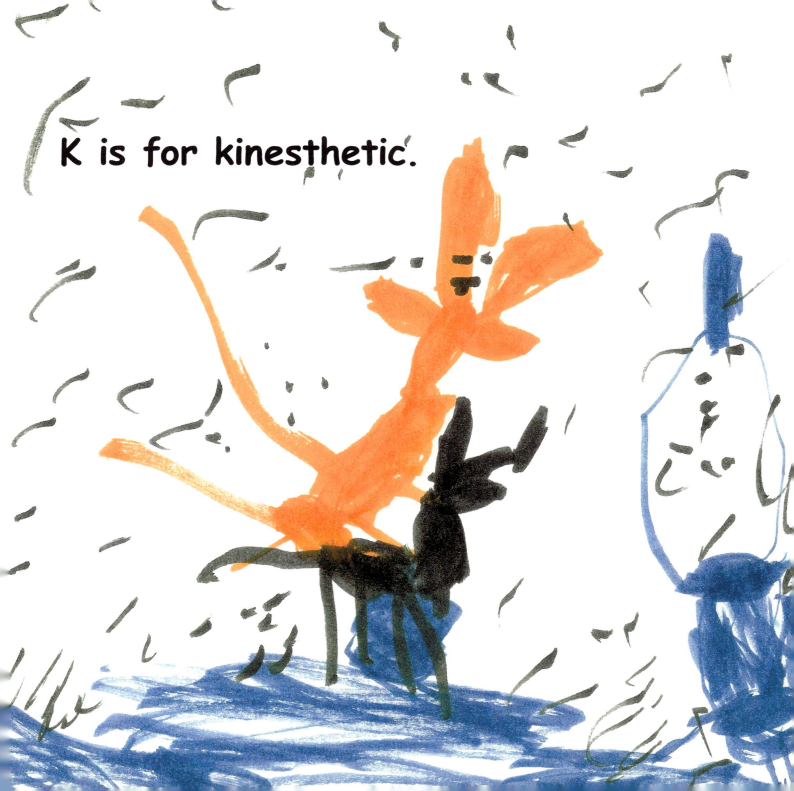
K is for kinesthetic.

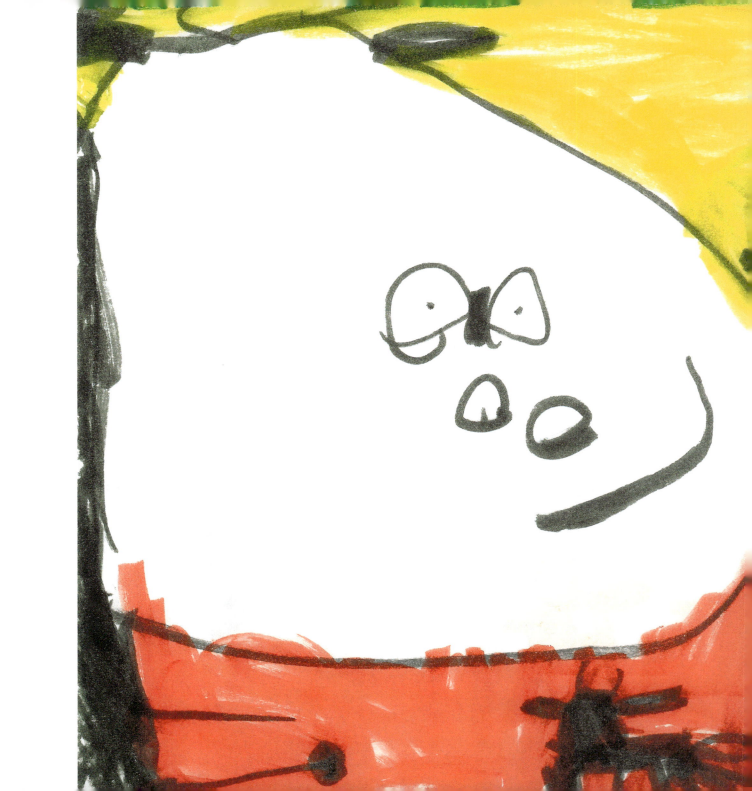

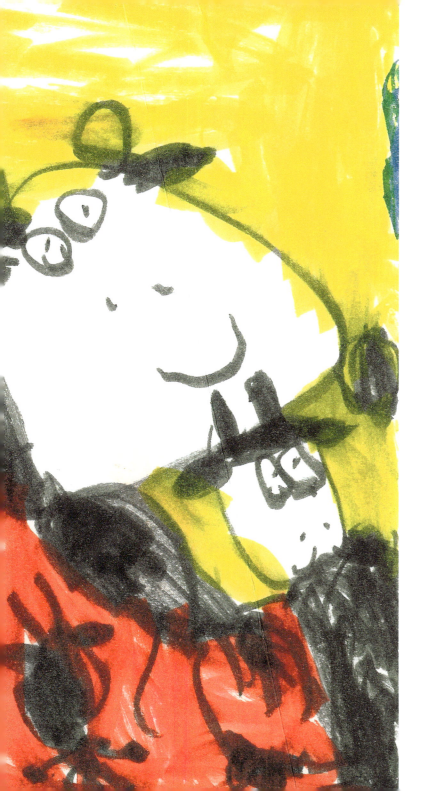

L is for love,
love, love.

M is Mom.
50 years ago the cause of autism was noted as "bad mothering". It's not your fault.

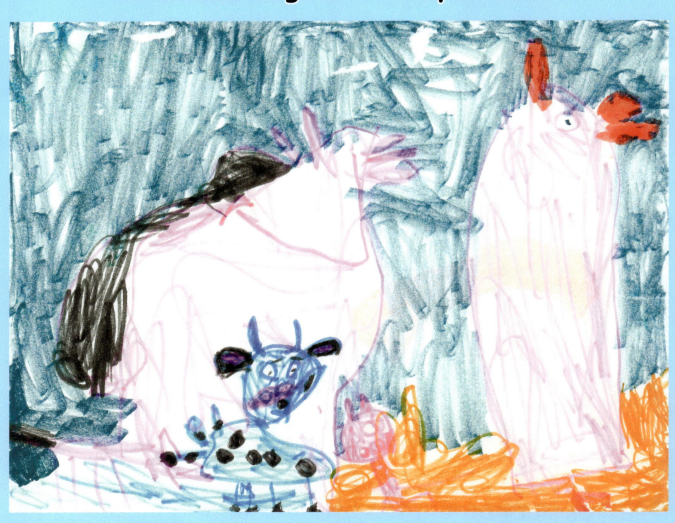

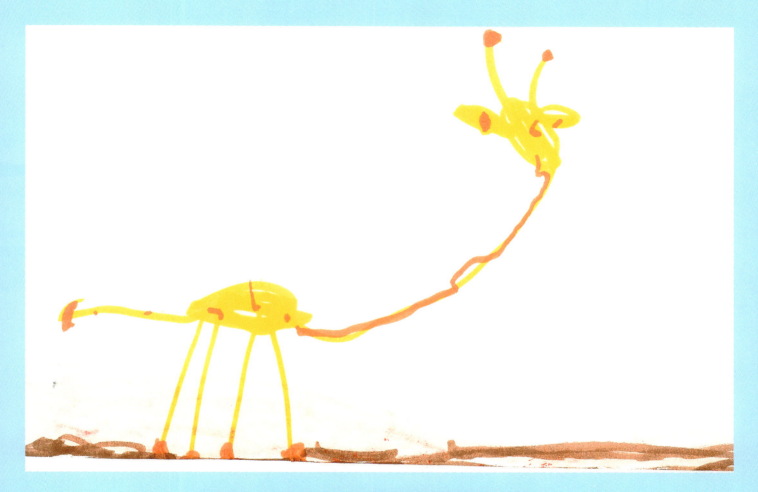

N is NUTRITION!

O is for over-diagnosing.

A small percentage of children are over-diagnosed with Autism Spectrum Disorder. Do your homework and do not drug your child.

and

Onset: Most austistic children develop normally until the age 18-22 mos.

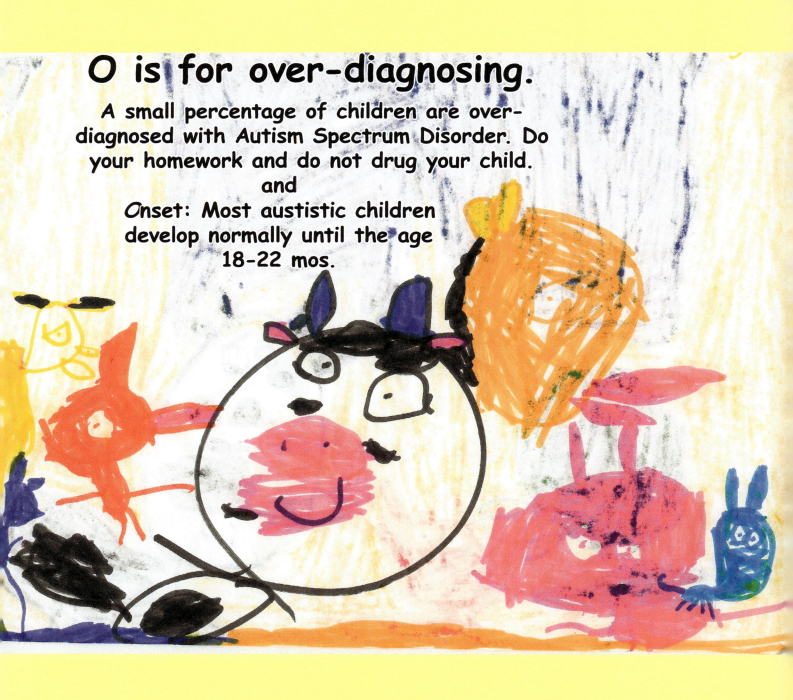

P is for...

Parents Helping Parents, patience, prayers and pottytraining, which usually doesn't happen until about age 6.

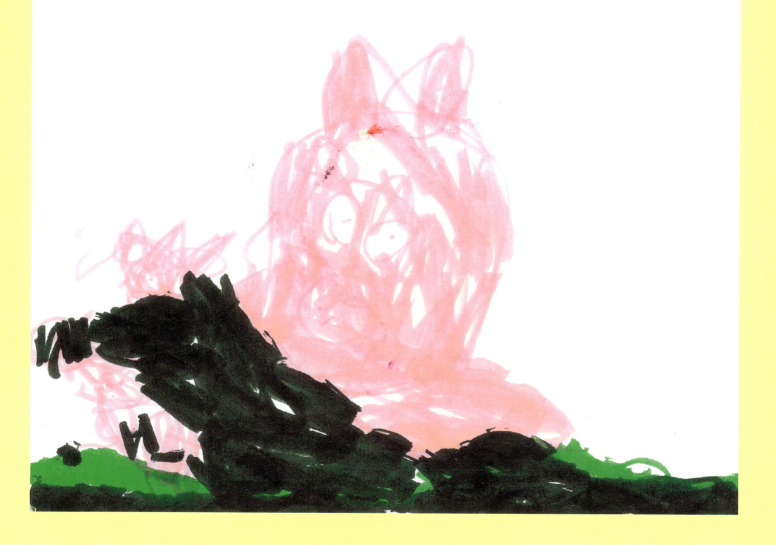

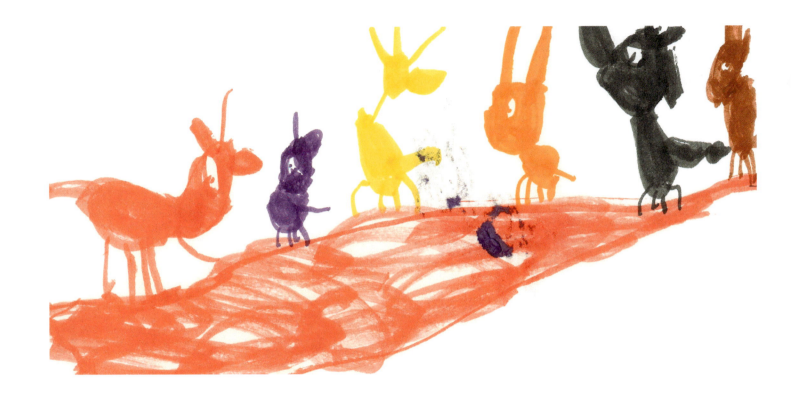

Q is for quiet.

The senses are typically overloaded creating a desire to withdraw.

R is for respect.

Not all autistic persons agree that they need to be "cured".

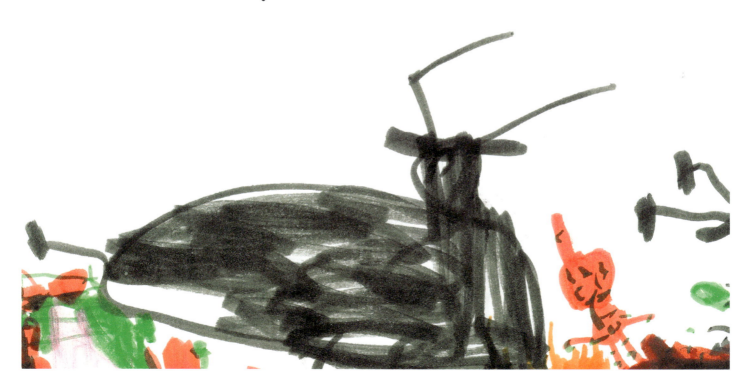

S is for speech.

One of the main hallmarks of autism is speech and language delay.

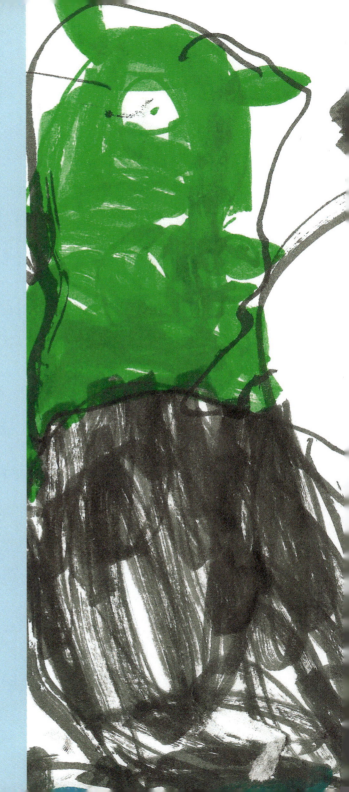

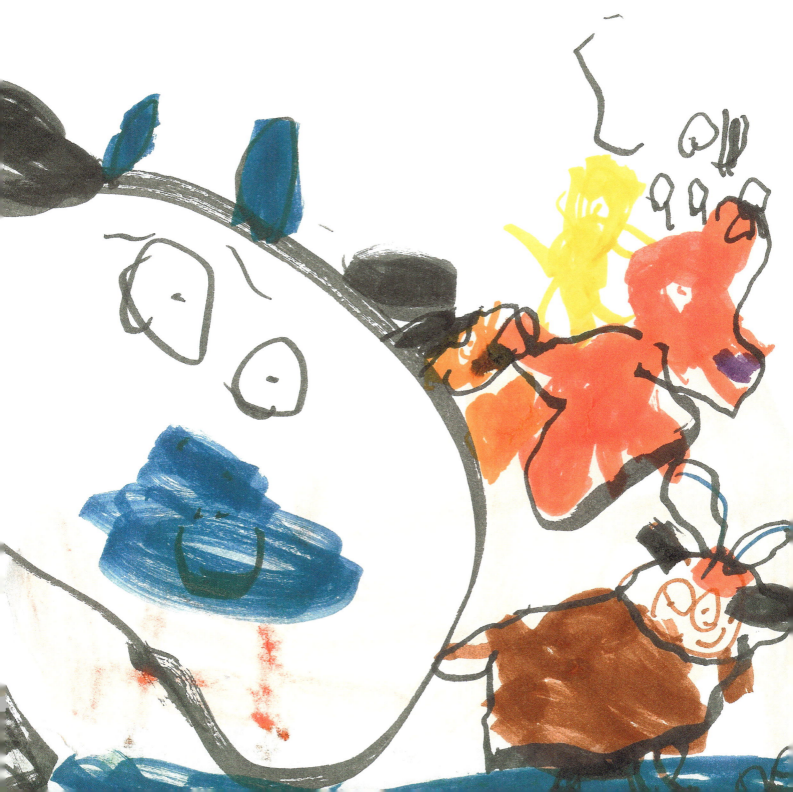

T is for tears, triumphs.

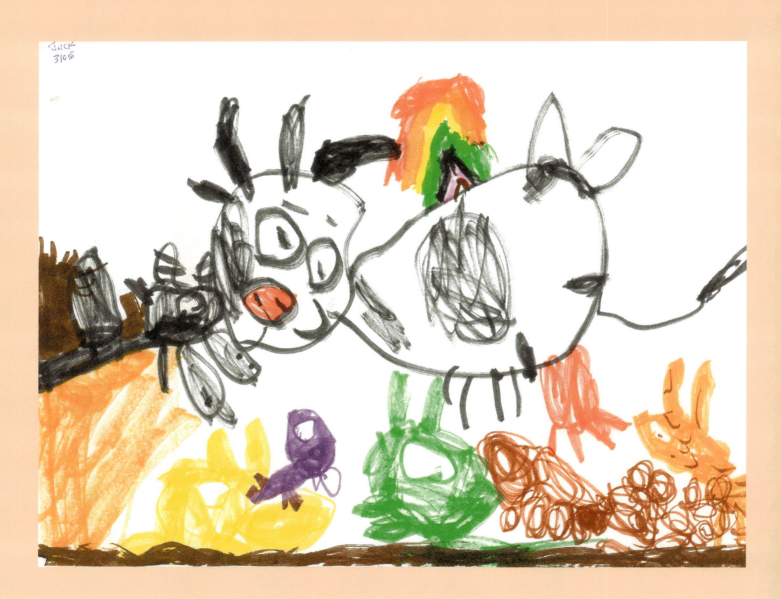

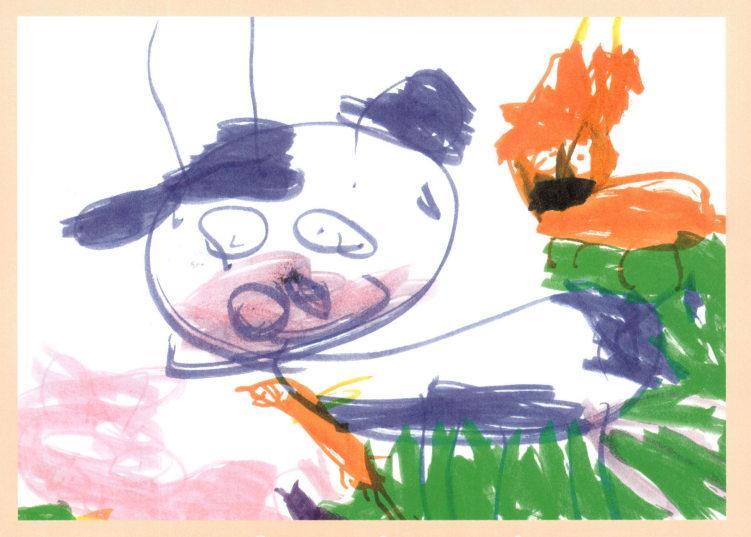

U is for Understanding.

High-functioning autistic people can usually understand everything going on around them and what you say, even if they don't respond.

V is for vaccinations —

Although not proven to cause autism, they are believed to worsen the effects of it.*

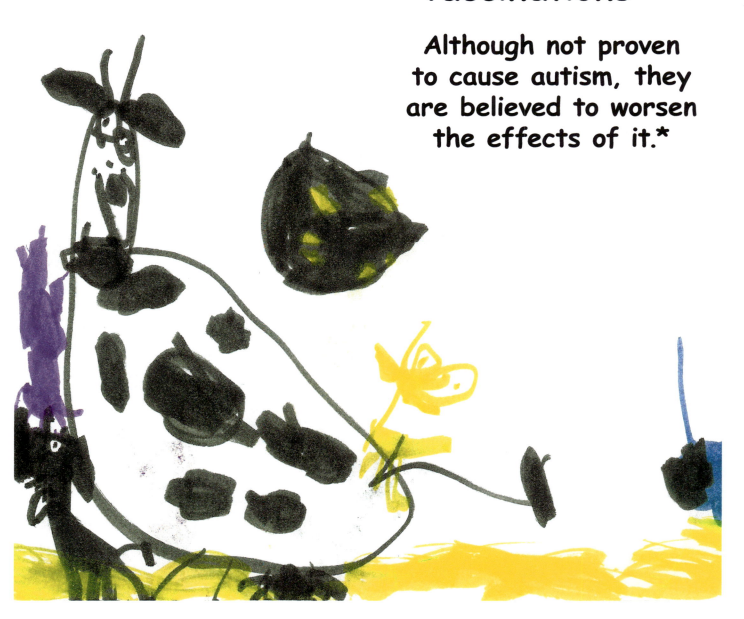

W is for wish, will power and wisdom.

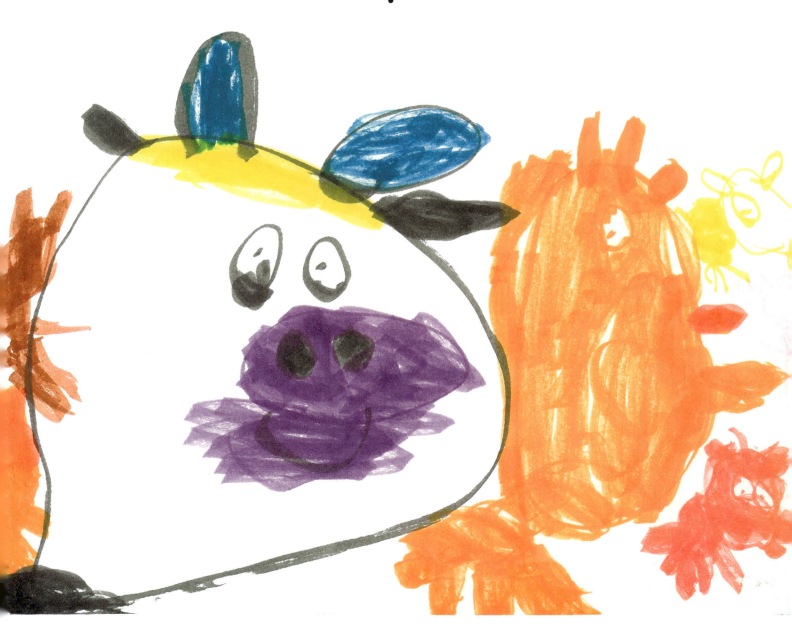

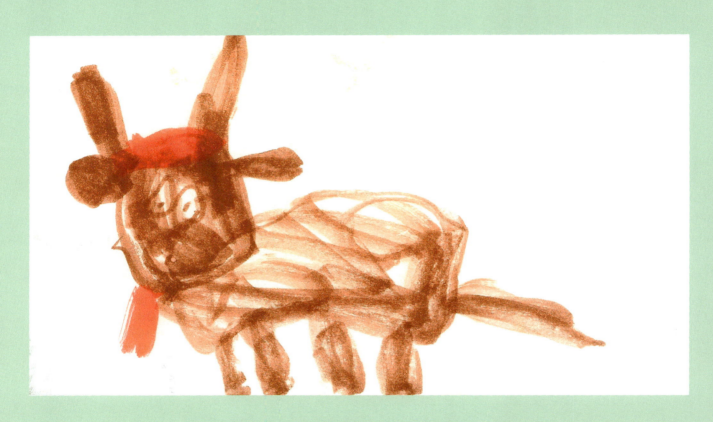

X is X-hausting!

Y is for yearning and yielding.

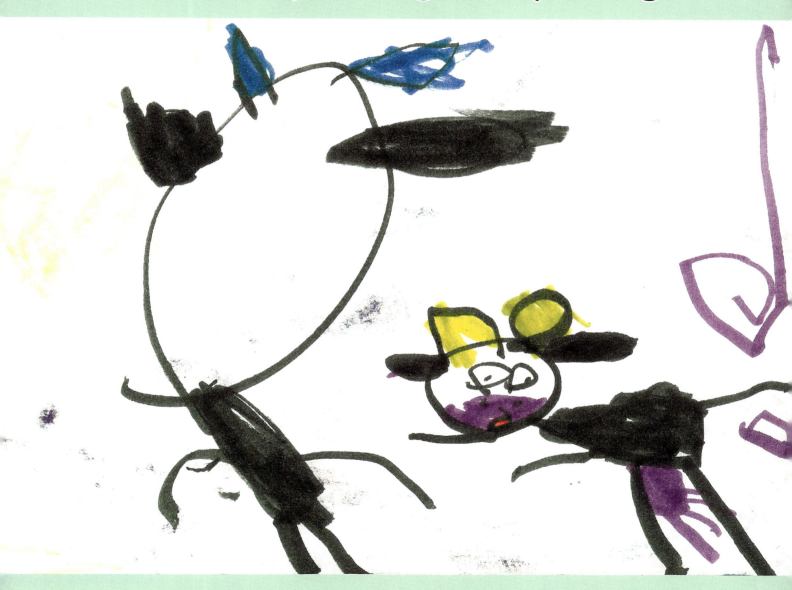

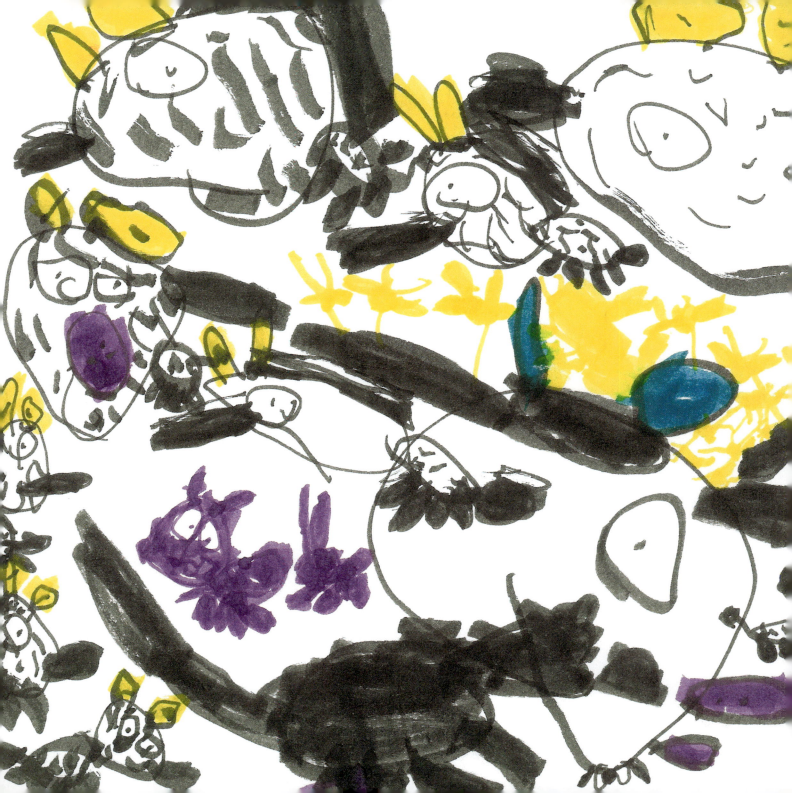

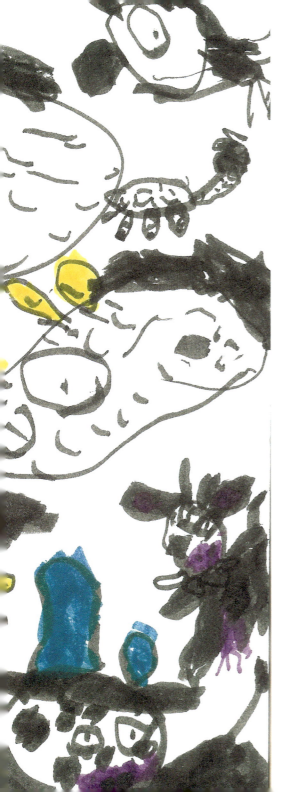

Z is for Zebra:

"A horse of a different stripe."

* A - Autism Society of Washington
* B - Autism Society of America
* E - Autism Education Network
* G - Autism Network for Dietary Intervention
* I - Autism Education Network
* J - Parents Helping Parents member
* V - Defeat Autism Now!

About the Author

A portion of the proceeds will go to the Autism Education Network and autism research. I originally put this book together with the drawings made by my 7-year old (autistic spectrum) son as a present for my husband's birthday.

As an author I have nothing previously published. I live in Los Gatos, California with my husband and three outstanding children.

Printed in the United States
1440LVUK00002B